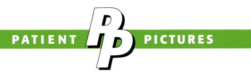

PATIENT PICTURES

Clinical drawings for your patients

Gastroenterology

Second edition

by
by Penny Neild MD FRCP
Consultant Gastroenterologist and Honorary Senior Lecturer
St George's Hospital
London, UK

Series Editor: J Richard Smith MD, FRCOG
Consultant Gynaecologist, Hammersmith and
Chelsea and Westminster Hospitals, London, UK
Honorary Consultant Gynaecologist, Royal Brompton Hospital, London, UK
Adjunct Associate Professor of Gynecology, New York University School of
Medicine, New York, USA

Illustrated by Dee McLean, MeDee Art, London, UK

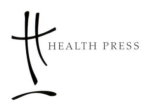

HEALTH PRESS

Oxford

Patient Pictures – Gastroenterology

First published 1997
Second edition August 2005

© 2005 in this edition Health Press Limited
Elizabeth House, Queen Street,
Abingdon, Oxford OX14 3LN, UK
Tel: +44 (0)1235 523233
Fax: +44 (0)1235 523238

Book orders can be placed by telephone or via the website.
For regional distributors or to order via the website, please go to:
www.patientpictures.com
For telephone orders, please call 01752 202301 (UK),
+44 1752 202301 (Europe), 800 266 5564 (USA) or 419 281 1802 (Canada).

Patient Pictures is a trademark of Health Press Limited.

A CIP catalogue record for this title is available from the British Library.

ISBN 1-903734-78-9

Neild P (Penny)
Patient Pictures – Gastroenterology/
Penny Neild

Medical illustrations by Dee McLean, London, UK.
Typesetting and page layout by Zed, Oxford, UK.
Printed by Quadrant Design and Print Solutions, Hertford, UK.

Printed with vegetable-oil-based inks on fully biodegradable and
recyclable paper manufactured from sustainable forests.

Reproduction authorization

The purchaser of this *Patient Pictures* series title is hereby authorized to reproduce, by photocopy only, any part of the pictorial and textual material contained in this work for non-profit, educational or patient education use. Photocopying for these purposes only is welcomed and free from further permission requirements from the publisher and free from any fee.

The reproduction of any material from this publication outside the guidelines above is strictly prohibited without the permission in writing of the publisher and is subject to minimum charges laid down by the Publishers Licensing Society Limited or its nominees.

Sarah Redston

Publisher, Health Press Limited, Oxford

Author's preface

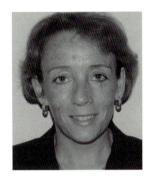

Gastroenterology encompasses many diseases and treatment procedures that are best explained, and easiest for patients to understand, when shown diagrammatically. Healthcare professionals often find themselves, perhaps in the midst of a busy surgery or clinic, attempting to illustrate their explanations to patients by sketching on a handy scrap of paper. Unfortunately, not all gastroenterologists are naturally gifted artists, and time is often limited, so the results can be confusing and frustrating for patient and doctor alike.

This book aims to provide clear, simple illustrations, supported by concise explanatory text, of some of the common gastroenterological conditions and procedures that are hard to describe in words alone. It is intended as a tool to aid healthcare professionals in their communication with patients, rather than as a comprehensive reference book.

I hope that you will find the book useful. If you have any suggestions for improvements, I and the Health Press team would be pleased to receive your feedback at post@healthpress.co.uk.

Penny Neild
St George's Hospital, London, UK

The gastrointestinal tract

- The digestive system – which is also known as the gastrointestinal tract – breaks down, digests and absorbs food, and removes solid waste from the body.

- The digestive system is a continuous muscular tube, anything from 5–9 metres (15–20 feet) long, which extends from the mouth to the anus. It consists of the gullet (oesophagus), stomach, small intestine, large intestine (colon), back passage (rectum) and anus.

- The oesophagus carries swallowed food to the stomach. In the stomach it is mixed with acidic juices to aid digestion. The food then gradually passes into the small intestine where digestion and absorption is completed with the aid of juices from the liver and pancreas. Any waste is transported to the large intestine and excreted via the rectum and anus.

- The liver, gall bladder, bile ducts and pancreas are important organs that are often considered as part of the digestive tract. They play a major role in the digestion of food and in the breakdown of potentially harmful waste substances.

- Common disorders that affect the digestive tract include infection and inflammation, muscular disturbances affecting the function of the tract, and cancers.

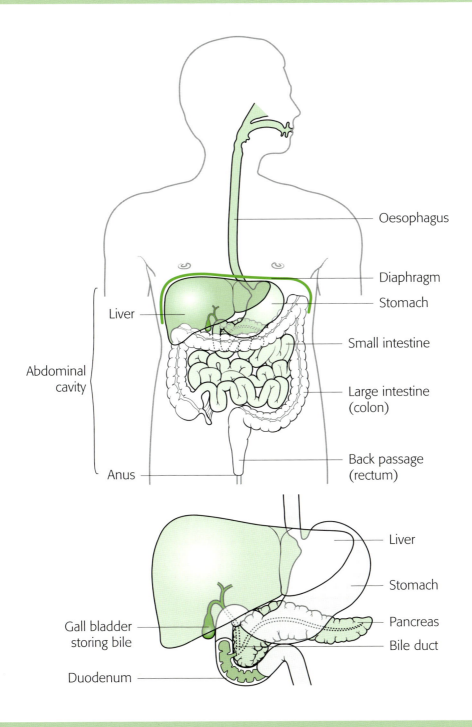

Oesophagus

Diaphragm

Stomach

Liver

Small intestine

Abdominal
cavity

Large intestine
(colon)

Back passage
(rectum)

Anus

Liver

Stomach

Pancreas

Gall bladder
storing bile

Bile duct

Duodenum

Hiatus hernia

- A hiatus hernia is caused by part of the stomach pushing up through a weakness in the diaphragm (the muscular sheet that lies underneath the lungs, separating the chest from the abdomen).

- In many people a hiatus hernia does not cause any symptoms and does not require any treatment.

- Hiatus hernia can lead to a backwards flow (reflux) of stomach contents or acid up into the oesophagus (gullet).

- Reflux causes heartburn, chest pain, waterbrash (sudden filling of the mouth with saliva) and regurgitation. These symptoms are worse when lying down, bending or straining after a meal.

- Hiatus hernia can be diagnosed using a barium swallow or endoscopy of the upper digestive tract.

- Reflux may be treated with lifestyle changes including losing weight, quitting smoking, eating smaller and more frequent meals, and avoiding eating immediately before going to bed or before strenuous exercise.

- Drugs may be used to treat reflux by reducing the amount of acid in the stomach or speeding up the rate at which food is passed out of the stomach into the intestines.

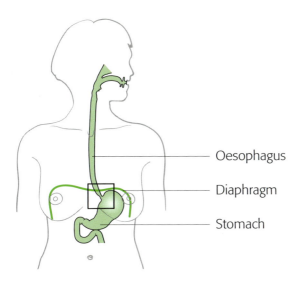

Oesophagus

Diaphragm

Stomach

Normal, strong diaphragm

Stomach pushes up through weakened diaphragm

Oesophagus

Gastro-oesophageal junction

Normal diaphragm

Weakened diaphragm

Stomach

Oesophagus

Gastro-oesophageal junction

Hiatus hernia

Stomach

Reflux of stomach contents

Gastro-oesophageal reflux, oesophagitis and Barrett's oesophagus

- 'Reflux' means the flow of the contents of the stomach and stomach acid backwards into the oesophagus (gullet).

- Reflux causes heartburn, chest pain, waterbrash (sudden filling of the mouth with saliva) and regurgitation. These symptoms are worse when lying down, bending or straining after a meal.

- A number of conditions can make reflux worse, including hiatus hernia, obesity, high alcohol intake, caffeine, large and/or fatty meals, and possibly smoking.

- Continual or repeated reflux can make the lower oesophagus inflamed (oesophagitis); this can cause stricture (narrowing) of the oesophagus. After several years, the lining of the oesophagus may change, a condition called Barrett's oesophagus. There is a very small possibility that it may eventually develop into cancer, so regular endoscopies may be recommended to monitor it.

- Gastro-oesophageal reflux can either be diagnosed by the doctor from your symptoms or by using endoscopy – examination of the intestine using a thin video 'telescope'. Occasionally, it is necessary to monitor the acidity of the oesophagus to confirm a diagnosis. This is done using an acidity meter in the form of a fine tube that is placed in the oesophagus for up to 24 hours.

- Reflux may be treated with drugs over the long term to reduce the amount of acid in the stomach. It is also important to avoid the factors that make the condition worse. Very occasionally, an operation may be required.

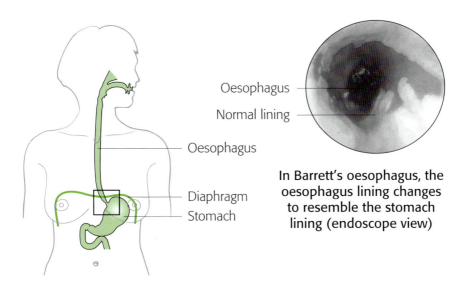

Oesophagus

Normal lining

In Barrett's oesophagus, the oesophagus lining changes to resemble the stomach lining (endoscope view)

Oesophagus

Diaphragm

Stomach

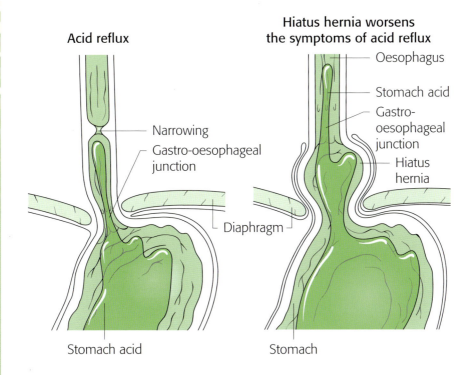

Acid reflux

Narrowing

Gastro-oesophageal junction

Stomach acid

Hiatus hernia worsens the symptoms of acid reflux

Oesophagus

Stomach acid

Gastro-oesophageal junction

Hiatus hernia

Diaphragm

Stomach

Oesophageal varices

- Oesophageal varices are veins in the oesophagus (gullet) that have become prominent and swollen because of liver disease. They are similar to varicose veins.

- As they enlarge and stretch, the swollen veins become fragile and likely to bleed if they are damaged, for example during swallowing, retching or vomiting.

- Oesophageal varices do not cause any symptoms until they bleed. When they bleed, you may vomit blood and pass dark red or black stools. If you lose a lot of blood, you will feel faint and weak.

- Some varices stop bleeding spontaneously, but because there is a risk of losing a lot of blood, an urgent and thorough hospital investigation is necessary. This usually involves examining the oesophagus using an endoscope (a thin video 'telescope').

- Oesophageal varices may be treated using an endoscope to inject the veins, or by placing a device like a rubber band on the veins to shrink them.

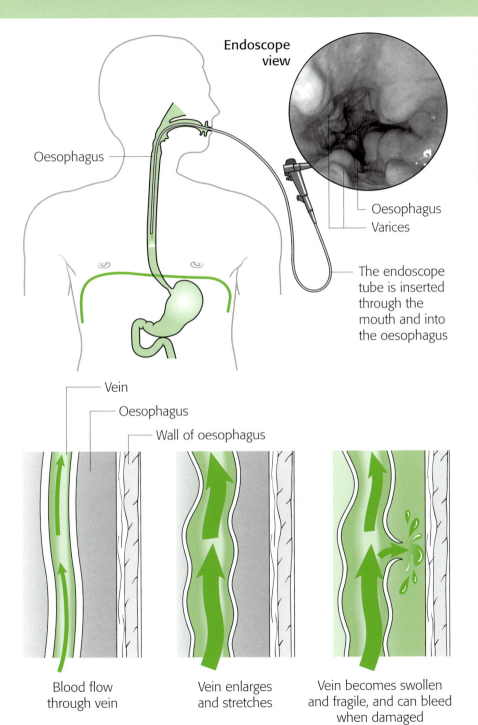

Endoscope view

Oesophagus

Oesophagus

Varices

The endoscope tube is inserted through the mouth and into the oesophagus

Vein

Oesophagus

Wall of oesophagus

Blood flow through vein

Vein enlarges and stretches

Vein becomes swollen and fragile, and can bleed when damaged

Oesophageal cancer

- The most common symptom of oesophageal cancer is difficulty in swallowing or the feeling that food is getting 'stuck' in the oesophagus (gullet).

- It is important to remember that these are also the symptoms of non-cancerous inflammation of the oesophagus (oesophagitis). Other symptoms of oesophageal cancer include painful swallowing, regurgitation of food and coughing, particularly when lying down.

- Oesophageal cancer can be detected during a barium swallow investigation, but endoscopy is necessary to confirm the diagnosis. Small tissue samples may be taken during endoscopy to determine the type of tumour.

- The treatment that is given will depend on the position and size of the cancer. It is not always possible to remove the cancer completely by surgery.

- An operation to remove the tumour may be considered if there is a good chance of removing the whole tumour, or if none of the above techniques is suitable for improving symptoms.

- Chemotherapy, radiotherapy (treatment with X-rays) or laser treatment can be used to reduce the size of the tumour, or an expandable mesh tube, called a stent, can be inserted into the oesophagus to keep it open and improve swallowing.

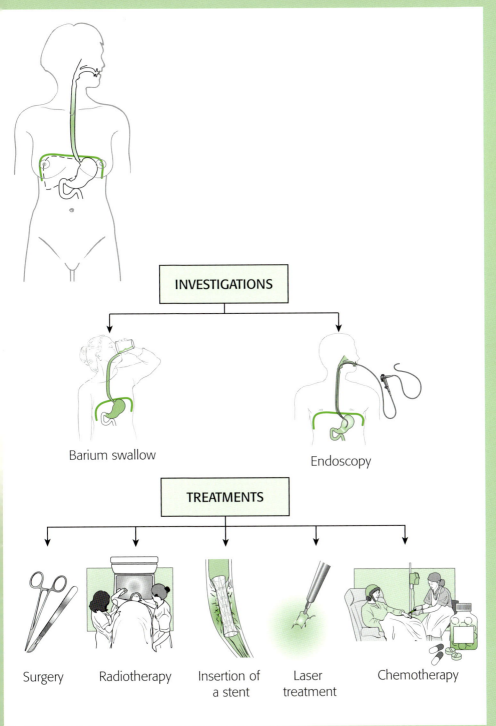

INVESTIGATIONS

Barium swallow

Endoscopy

TREATMENTS

Surgery

Radiotherapy

Insertion of
a stent

Laser
treatment

Chemotherapy

Peptic ulcer

- A peptic ulcer is a wound in the lining of the stomach or duodenum caused by the acid in the digestive juices. It is similar to a mouth ulcer.

- A typical symptom of peptic ulcer is a deep aching pain in the upper part of the abdomen, just below the breastbone, that may be relieved by eating or by taking antacid tablets. The pain tends to occur several times a day and lasts for 15 to 60 minutes. It may also occur at night.

- Drugs such as aspirin can cause peptic ulcers, as can smoking. Peptic ulcers occur more commonly in some families than others, but this may be because of shared environmental factors, such as diet, rather than a genetic tendency.

- About 40% of people are infected with the bacterium *Helicobacter pylori*, which usually causes no symptoms, but increases the risk of development of peptic ulcers.

- Treatment of peptic ulcer involves avoiding certain drugs, stopping smoking and treatment of any *Helicobacter pylori* infection. Medicine to stop the stomach from producing acid can be prescribed if symptoms persist.

- There are various ways of detecting the bacterium, including a breath test and a blood test. Occasionally, it may be necessary to examine the intestine with an endoscope (a thin video 'telescope') and to take a small tissue sample (biopsy).

- *Helicobacter pylori* infection can be cured with a combination of antibiotics taken for 1–2 weeks.

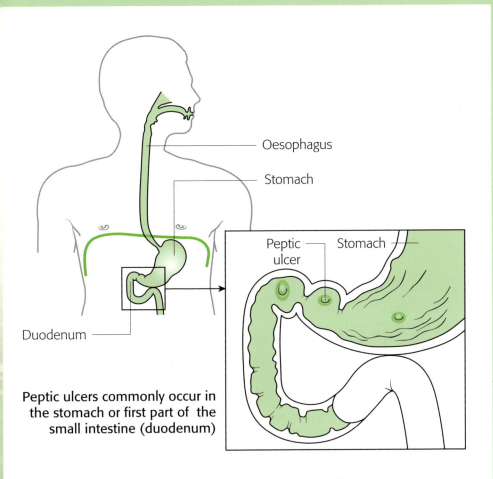

Oesophagus

Stomach

Peptic ulcer

Stomach

Duodenum

Peptic ulcers commonly occur in the stomach or first part of the small intestine (duodenum)

Endoscopy

Barium meal before X-ray

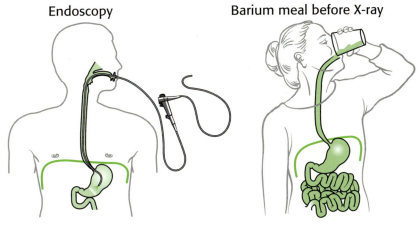

Cancer of the stomach (gastric cancer)

- Symptoms of stomach cancer are often mild and include indigestion, weight loss and loss of appetite. It is important to remember that these symptoms are also common in non-cancerous disorders of the digestive system.

- The cancer can be diagnosed using barium meal or endoscopy of the upper digestive system – examination of the intestine using a thin video 'telescope'. Small tissue samples may be taken during endoscopy (biopsy) to confirm the type of tumour.

- Treatment will depend on the size and position of the tumour, and whether or not the cancer has spread to other parts of the body.

- It may be possible to remove some or all of the cancer in a large operation which involves removal of all or most of the stomach and of the local lymph glands. After the operation your stomach will be smaller and so you will have to eat more frequent, small meals.

- Other treatment options include chemotherapy and, sometimes, radiotherapy (treatment with X-rays), which may be used together with surgery.

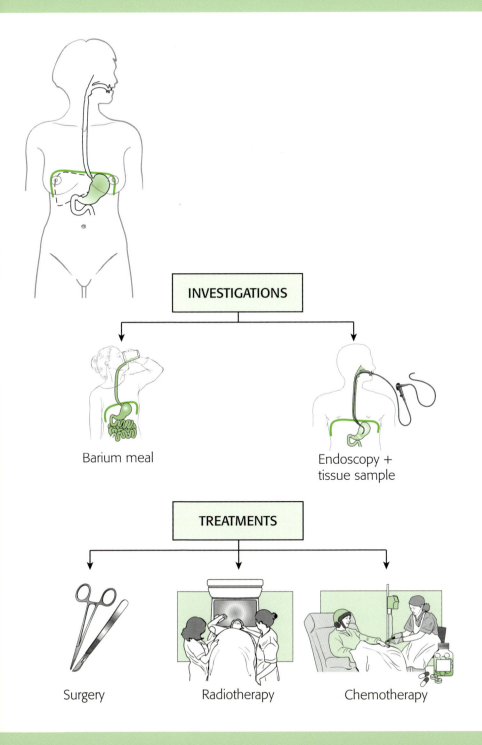

INVESTIGATIONS

Barium meal

Endoscopy +
tissue sample

TREATMENTS

Surgery

Radiotherapy

Chemotherapy

Coeliac disease

- Coeliac disease is caused by an allergic reaction to gluten, a protein which is present in food containing wheat, barley, rye or oats. Although it is a lifelong condition, it is most commonly diagnosed in adults.

- Symptoms of coeliac disease include loss of weight, a bloated abdomen, diarrhoea with pale stools, anaemia, general weakness and mouth ulcers. These symptoms are caused by poor absorption of vitamins and nutrients through the intestine.

- Coeliac disease can be diagnosed using blood tests, but it is often necessary to examine a small piece of tissue from the small intestine to confirm the diagnosis. This is obtained by endoscopy (examination of the intestine using a video 'telescope').

- Coeliac disease is treated by following a special diet. Foods to avoid include those made from wheat flour, such as bread, cakes, biscuits and pastries, and those containing rye, barley or oats. People often notice that their symptoms improve within days of starting a gluten-free diet.

- Coeliac disease is a lifelong condition, but you can stay in good health if you continue to follow the gluten-free diet. Gluten-free foods are available on prescription, and you will receive advice from a dietician.

- The Coeliac Society (www.coeliac.co.uk; 01494 437278) also provides useful information on foods that must be avoided and those that can be eaten freely, including food available in the major supermarket chains.

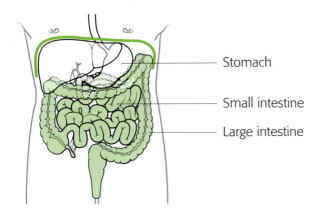

Stomach

Small intestine

Large intestine

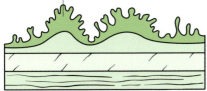

Finger-like villi help absorb nutrients and vitamins

Normal intestinal lining

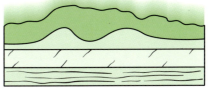

Inflamed, eroded lining cannot absorb nutrients

Intestinal lining in coeliac disease

Foods to eat freely

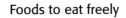

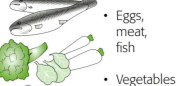

- Milk & dairy products

- Eggs, meat, fish

- Vegetables

- Fruit

- Rice, pulses

Foods to avoid

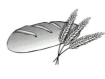
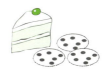

- Bread (made from wheat flour)

- Normal cakes and biscuits

- Pastries and pies

Gallstones

- Gallstones of various sizes and shapes may form in the gall bladder. They are made up of cholesterol, calcium and bile salts. The stones can be seen by ultrasound or endoscopic retrograde cholangiopancreatography.

- Most gallstones remain in the gall bladder and do not cause any symptoms. Symptoms occur when the stones move and get stuck in the neck of the gall bladder or in the bile duct.

- Inflammation of the gall bladder (acute cholecystitis) caused by gallstones can cause severe abdominal pain that comes on suddenly and is accompanied by wind and nausea. You may have to be admitted to hospital for treatment. Symptoms normally go away spontaneously, but it may be necessary to remove the gall bladder in order to prevent a recurrence. This does not have a major effect on your ability to digest food.

- If gallstones are blocking the bile duct, you may have severe abdominal pain (biliary colic). Symptoms may clear up without treatment if the stones move into the intestine. An endoscopic examination is usually performed to check that no stones are left in the bile ducts and to remove any still there.

- If the blocked bile duct is infected, the pain may be accompanied by vomiting, jaundice and fever (cholangitis). This requires antibiotics and, usually, admission to hospital.

- Gallstones may cause chronic (persistent) cholecystitis. Recurring bouts of abdominal pain are common, and you may also feel pain in your back or right shoulder. Treatment involves an operation to remove the gall bladder.

- In the majority of patients the gall bladder can be removed using laparoscopy (keyhole surgery). Occasionally, conventional surgery is required.

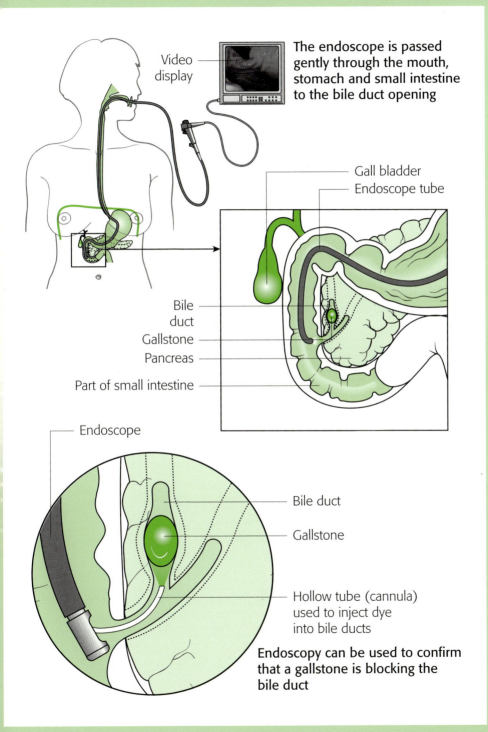

Video display

The endoscope is passed gently through the mouth, stomach and small intestine to the bile duct opening

Gall bladder

Endoscope tube

Bile duct

Gallstone

Pancreas

Part of small intestine

Endoscope

Bile duct

Gallstone

Hollow tube (cannula) used to inject dye into bile ducts

Endoscopy can be used to confirm that a gallstone is blocking the bile duct

Chronic pancreatitis

- Chronic (persistent) pancreatitis is continuous inflammation of the pancreas. The pancreas is a gland linked to the liver and small intestine; it secretes digestive enzymes and insulin.

- Chronic pancreatitis is more common in men than women, and may occur as a result of long-term excess alcohol intake. Occasionally it may be due to gallstones.

- The main symptom is persistent abdominal pain, which may also be felt in the back. You may lose appetite and weight, and suffer from diarrhoea.

- Chronic pancreatitis is usually diagnosed using ultrasound and/or endoscopic examination (ERCP). Occasionally the diagnosis can be made from a simple abdominal X-ray.

- The condition is treated using painkillers. If you have diarrhoea, which is caused by poor digestion of food, pancreatic enzyme supplements may also be used. You should also avoid alcohol.

- The pain usually lessens with time, provided you avoid alcohol permanently.

- An operation to remove part of the pancreas is sometimes required if the pain is severe and does not improve with medical treatments.

- Up to 30% of patients who suffer from chronic pancreatitis as a result of long-term excess alcohol intake develop diabetes.

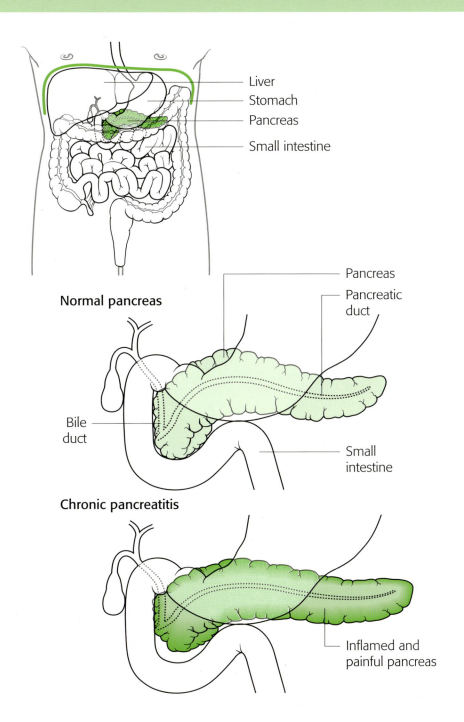

Liver
Stomach
Pancreas
Small intestine

Normal pancreas

Pancreas
Pancreatic duct

Bile duct

Small intestine

Chronic pancreatitis

Inflamed and painful pancreas

Pancreatic cancer

- Symptoms of pancreatic cancer are often mild and non-specific, such as tiredness, lack of energy, weight loss and vomiting. Jaundice, skin irritation and abdominal pain occur later in the disease.

- The cancer can be detected using blood tests and ultrasound or CT scans. A tissue sample (biopsy) is also taken, either through the skin using ultrasound or CT to guide the procedure, or using an endoscope (a flexible video 'telescope'). The sample is examined in the laboratory to confirm the diagnosis.

- Treatment depends upon the size and position of the tumour. An operation to remove the cancer is sometimes possible.

- Radiotherapy (treatment with X-rays) and chemotherapy are other treatment options.

- If the cancer blocks the bile ducts on the pancreas, jaundice and itching can result. The bile ducts can be unblocked either by inserting a stent (a small plastic or metal tube) or by creating a bypass surgically.

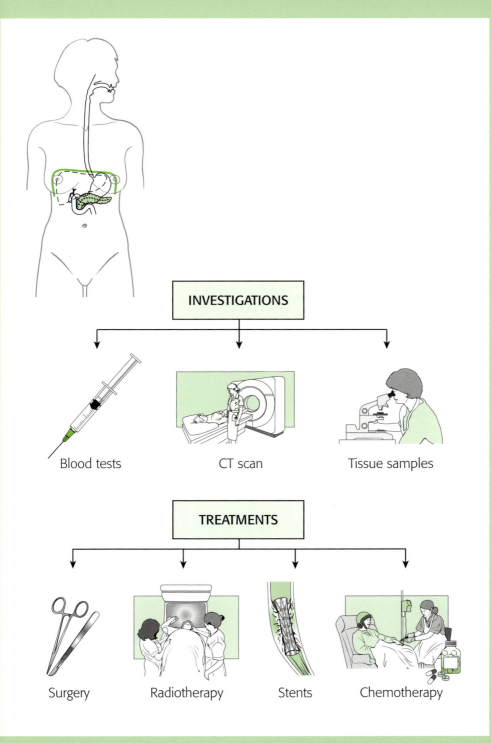

INVESTIGATIONS

Blood tests

CT scan

Tissue samples

TREATMENTS

Surgery

Radiotherapy

Stents

Chemotherapy

Cirrhosis of the liver

- In cirrhosis, the liver tissue thickens and scars, the flow of blood through the liver is reduced, and the liver's ability to make proteins and remove toxic waste products from the body is lessened.

- The two most common causes of liver cirrhosis are excessive alcohol intake and viral hepatitis, but any chronic liver disease can cause long-term damage.

- Symptoms of liver cirrhosis include general tiredness, lack of energy, loss of sex drive and skin discoloration.

- When the liver has been severely damaged, complications may occur. Oesophageal and gastric varices (veins that have become prominent and swollen because of reduced blood flow) can develop and they may burst, causing serious blood loss.

- Varices may be treated using an endoscope (a flexible video 'telescope') to inject a medicine or place a band on the veins to shrink them. Alternatively, an operation may be carried out to bypass the damaged liver and reduce the pressure on the blood vessels.

- Another possible complication of cirrhosis is ascites, the build-up of fluid in the abdomen, causing bloating and discomfort. Medicine can be taken to reduce the fluid retention, or the fluid can be drained away using a fine, sterile tube.

- If the liver is severely damaged, a transplant operation may be required.

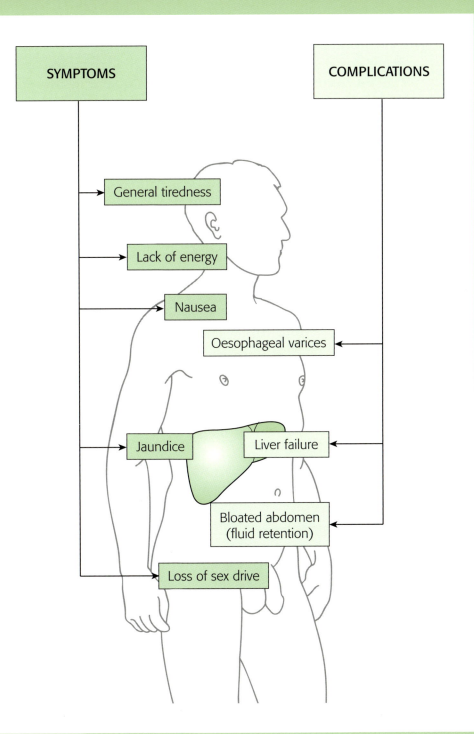

SYMPTOMS

COMPLICATIONS

General tiredness

Lack of energy

Nausea

Oesophageal varices

Jaundice

Liver failure

Bloated abdomen
(fluid retention)

Loss of sex drive

Irritable bowel syndrome

- Irritable bowel syndrome is a very common condition caused by abnormal contractions of the muscles in the large intestine and increased sensitivity of the bowel to the presence of gas and movement. It appears to be made worse by stress.

- Symptoms include recurring, cramp-like or colicky abdominal pain and irregular bowel movements, from diarrhoea to constipation.

- The symptoms are not usually severe, and may disappear without treatment for periods ranging from days to years.

- Irritable bowel syndrome can usually be diagnosed without specialized investigations, but if there is any doubt, the colon can be examined using barium enema or colonoscopy.

- Modifying your diet can relieve symptoms. There are no specific foods that make irritable bowel syndrome worse in everyone, so most patients adjust their diet according to their own experiences or with help from dieticians.

- If symptoms persist, your doctor may prescribe bulking agents, or else tablets that alter the movement of the bowel, prevent muscle spasm or reduce the bowel's sensitivity to the presence of gas and to muscle movements.

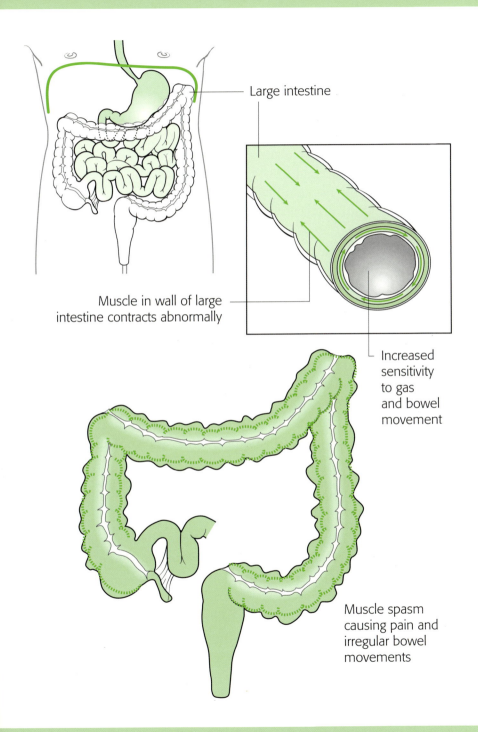

Large intestine

Muscle in wall of large intestine contracts abnormally

Increased sensitivity to gas and bowel movement

Muscle spasm causing pain and irregular bowel movements

Crohn's disease

- Crohn's disease is a chronic (persistent) disease that involves inflammation of the digestive tract. The disease varies in severity.

- Symptoms vary according to the part of the digestive tract that is affected, but usually include colicky abdominal pain, diarrhoea and weight loss. The disease may also cause arthritis of the back and large joints, inflamed eyes, skin rashes and inflammation of the biliary tract and liver.

- Barium meal, barium follow through or barium enema may be used to diagnose the disease and colonoscopy is often carried out so that a small tissue sample can be obtained for examination in the laboratory to confirm the diagnosis.

- Treatment depends upon the site of the disease, but includes corticosteroids and drugs to reduce the inflammation. The drugs can be given as an enema if the large intestine and rectum are affected.

- Dietary adjustments and vitamin and mineral supplements can also help. When the digestive system is inflamed, a specialized diet may be prescribed consisting of foods that require very little digestion before being absorbed.

- Patients have regular check-ups as outpatients in hospital to monitor their condition. If you have severe symptoms, you may be admitted to hospital for treatment.

- Occasionally, when symptoms cannot be controlled by drug treatment, it is necessary to remove the inflamed part of the intestine in an operation.

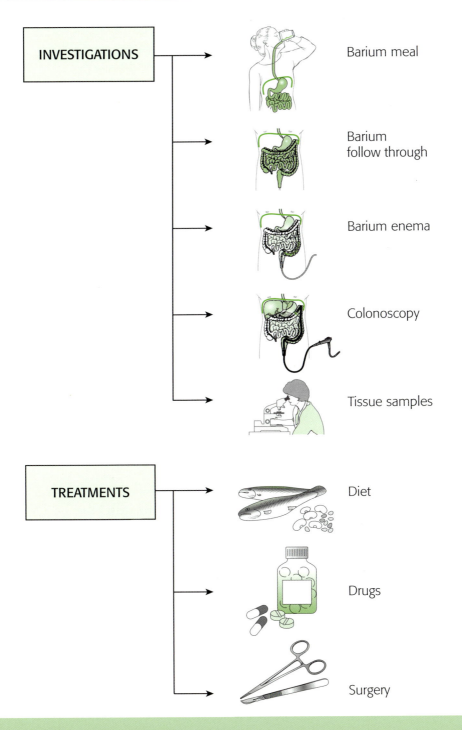

INVESTIGATIONS

Barium meal

Barium follow through

Barium enema

Colonoscopy

Tissue samples

TREATMENTS

Diet

Drugs

Surgery

Ulcerative colitis

- Ulcerative colitis is a chronic (persistent) disease caused by inflammation of the colon and rectum (back passage); it varies in severity and extent.

- People with ulcerative colitis pass frequent loose stools, which may contain blood and mucus. They may also have abdominal cramps, arthritis in the back and the large joints, inflamed eyes, skin rashes and inflammation of the biliary tract and liver.

- Diagnosis is made by colonoscopy (or sigmoidoscopy) and by examining a tissue sample taken during the colonoscopy.

- Treatment involves drugs to reduce the inflammation and, for severe symptoms, corticosteroids. The drugs can be given as an enema if only the lower large intestine and rectum are affected. Drug doses are reduced between attacks, but you need to keep taking them to prevent recurrence of the disease.

- Patients have regular check-ups as outpatients in hospital to monitor their condition. If you have severe symptoms, you may be admitted to hospital for treatment.

- Occasionally, if symptoms cannot be controlled with drugs, it is necessary to remove the colon. If this is the case, the surgeon will make the end of the remaining small bowel into a false rectum or into an artificial opening on the surface of the abdomen (ileostomy).

- Ten years after diagnosis, patients with ulcerative colitis should have annual colonoscopy investigations because in some cases there is an increased risk of cancer of the colon. Regular check-ups will allow early diagnosis and treatment of this disease.

INVESTIGATIONS

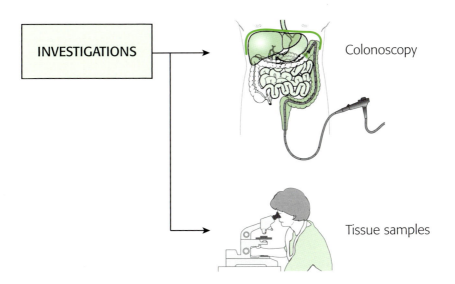

Colonoscopy

Tissue samples

TREATMENTS

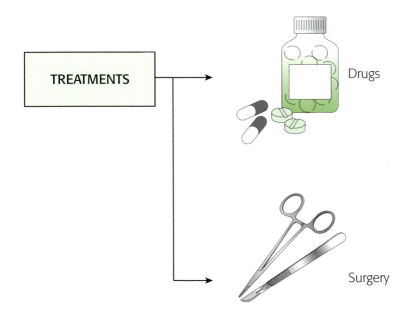

Drugs

Surgery

Diverticular disease

- A diverticulum is a small pouch or 'sac' that is formed when the lining of the intestine pushes through a weak area in its wall.

- Diverticular disease is associated with a diet that is low in fibre. It is common in older people, especially those over 70 years old, but in Western societies it is increasingly seen in younger people too.

- In many people, diverticular disease does not produce any symptoms, and it is usually diagnosed by chance when a barium enema or colonoscopy examination is carried out to investigate another condition (for example, constipation or bleeding from the rectum).

- A small number of patients may suffer persistent or colicky pain and may also find they are passing small, pellet-like stools.

- These symptoms can be relieved by increasing the amount of fibre in the diet, which reduces the amount of work that the colon needs to do to move waste material through the intestine.

- Rarely, complications may develop, such as infection or perforation of a diverticulum. These cause more severe pain and fever, with bleeding from the rectum (back passage). If this occurs, you will be given antibiotics and may have to be admitted to hospital. An operation may also be needed to remove the damaged part of the intestine, and this may mean you have to have a colostomy.

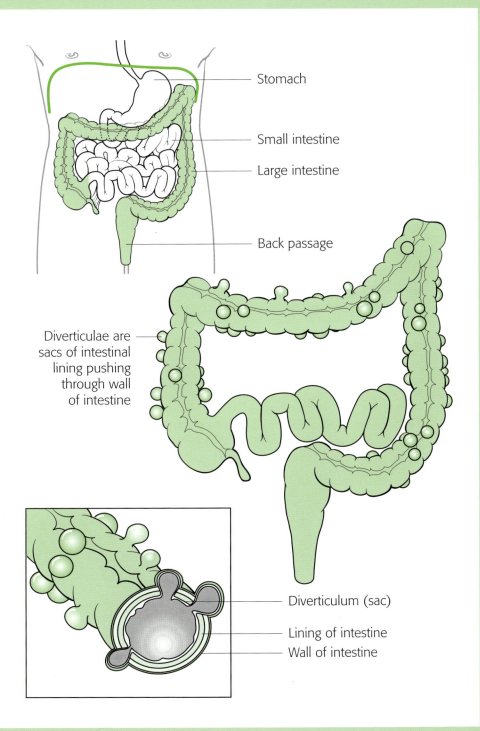

Stomach

Small intestine

Large intestine

Back passage

Diverticulae are sacs of intestinal lining pushing through wall of intestine

Diverticulum (sac)

Lining of intestine
Wall of intestine

Colorectal polyps

- Colorectal polyps are non-cancerous growths that form on the inner wall of the large intestine and rectum (back passage). They are extremely common, particularly in older people.

- It is not clear what causes polyps, but there is a rare condition that can be inherited, in which many polyps form in young patients from childhood onwards. Screening of children who have relatives with this condition is available from 12 years of age.

- Colorectal polyps may not produce any symptoms, although they can cause bleeding from the rectum, abdominal pain, or a change in bowel movements.

- Polyps can be diagnosed using a barium enema investigation or colonoscopy with a colonoscope (a flexible video 'telescope').

- Once diagnosed, colorectal polyps should be removed, because there is a small risk that they may eventually become cancerous. Polyps are usually removed during colonoscopy, but occasionally an operation is required.

- Polyps are removed by colonoscopy using a small instrument that is passed down a colonoscope. The polyp is trapped in a 'snare' and then separated painlessly from the wall of the intestine, using an electric current to seal the blood vessels.

- After removal, the polyp will be examined in the laboratory to check for any abnormalities. You will be asked to return to hospital for a check-up every few years to make sure that no new polyps have formed.

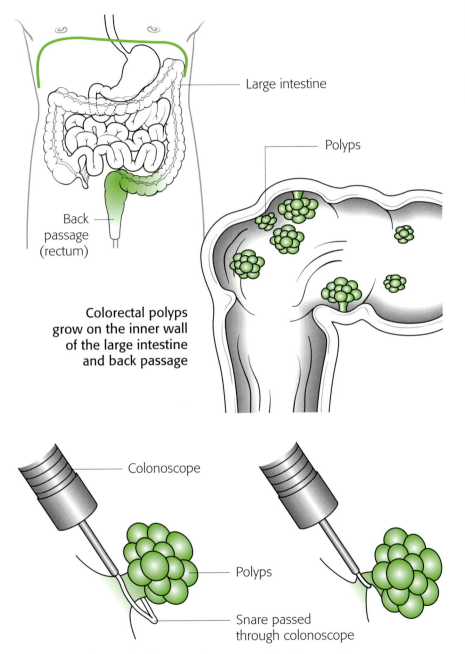

Large intestine

Polyps

Back passage (rectum)

Colorectal polyps grow on the inner wall of the large intestine and back passage

Colonoscope

Polyps

Snare passed through colonoscope

Colorectal polyps can be removed using a colonoscope

Cancer of the colon

- Cancer of the colon often develops from a colorectal polyp, which is a non-cancerous growth on the inner wall of the large intestine and rectum. The tendency for polyps to become cancerous may be inherited.

- Symptoms include a change in your normal bowel movements, with either diarrhoea or constipation. You may see some blood in your stools, or feel that you have not finished after a bowel movement.

- Diagnosis is usually made after a barium enema or colonoscopy investigation. A small piece of tissue may be removed (biopsy) and examined in the laboratory to confirm the type of cancer.

- An operation is usually needed to remove the cancer. If it is not possible to join the colon back together again after taking out the growth, a temporary or permanent artificial opening (called a stoma) for the colon will be made on the abdomen (colostomy). If this is likely, you will be given counselling before the operation and help afterwards, until you are able to look after the stoma yourself.

- If the cancer is too widespread for surgery, treatment options include radiotherapy and chemotherapy.

- Radiotherapy and chemotherapy may also be used with surgery to increase the likelihood that all the cancer cells will be destroyed, and that you will be cured.

- After your operation, you will be asked to return to hospital for colonoscopy every 2–3 years to make sure that the cancer does not return, and to remove any new polyps that form.

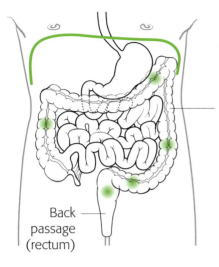

Tinted circles show possible sites of cancer

Large intestine (colon)

Back passage (rectum)

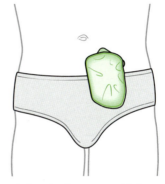

Abdominal stoma with bag

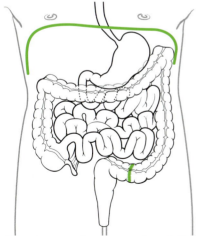

The tumour is removed and the colon is joined back together

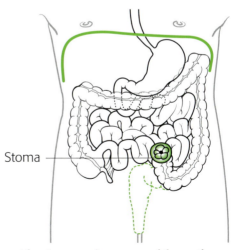

Stoma

The tumour is removed from the rectum and a 'stoma' created as an artificial opening on the abdomen

Haemorrhoids

- Haemorrhoids, or 'piles', are swollen fleshy pads filled with veins. They occur just inside the rectum (back passage) or on the anus.

- Haemorrhoids are very common, and often run in the family. They may be associated with constipation or straining during bowel movements, and often occur for the first time during pregnancy.

- Symptoms include bleeding from the rectum, usually after a bowel motion (blood may be seen on toilet paper), pain in the rectum, particularly when a stool is being passed, and collapse of the haemorrhoids out of the rectum when passing a stool. The haemorrhoids may return into the body spontaneously, but may need to be pushed back gently with a finger.

- Haemorrhoids inside the rectum may be diagnosed by the doctor gently examining your rectum with a finger, or using a proctoscope (an instrument that enables the inside of the rectum to be seen).

- Haemorrhoids can usually be treated in the outpatient department. You will either be given an injection via the rectum that will cause the swellings to shrink, or the swellings will be reduced in size by placing small elastic bands over their base. These procedures are painless, although you may feel some discomfort.

- Large or more complicated haemorrhoids may have to be removed in an operation.

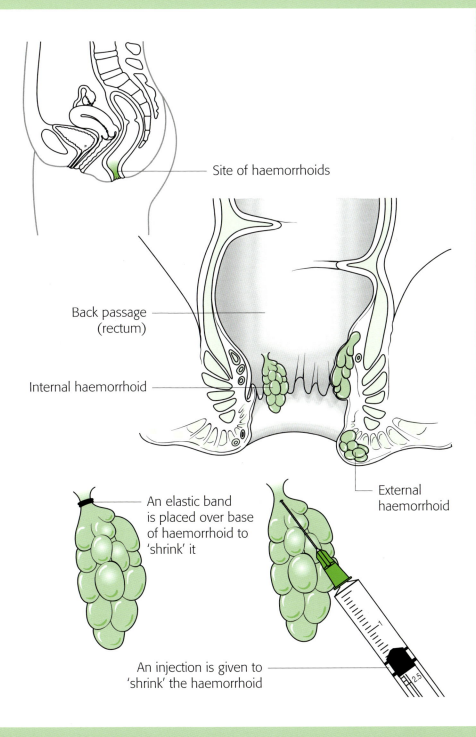

Site of haemorrhoids

Back passage
(rectum)

Internal haemorrhoid

External
haemorrhoid

An elastic band
is placed over base
of haemorrhoid to
'shrink' it

An injection is given to
'shrink' the haemorrhoid

Endoscopy of the upper gastrointestinal tract

- Endoscopy is the examination of the inside of the digestive system using a flexible video 'telescope' called an endoscope. Endoscopy enables the specialist to look inside you without surgery.

- Endoscopy of the upper digestive system is used to look at the oesophagus (gullet), the stomach and the first part of the small intestine. It is usually used to investigate symptoms such as difficulty in swallowing, heartburn, abdominal pain and vomiting.

- You will be asked not to eat or drink for at least 6 hours before the procedure to ensure that your stomach is empty.

- Before the procedure, you may be given an injection of sedative, which will cause drowsiness but will not send you completely to sleep. Alternatively, local anaesthetic may be sprayed onto the back of your throat.

- The feeling of the endoscopy tube at the back of your throat may be uncomfortable, but it will not affect your breathing.

- If any areas appear abnormal, tiny pieces of tissue may be painlessly removed for further examination. This is called a biopsy. You should have the results within a fortnight.

- The procedure usually takes no longer than 5–10 minutes, and you will be able to go home the same day. If you are given a sedative, someone should accompany you home, as the effects of the injection may last for several hours.

- If a local anaesthetic spray is used, you should not eat or drink for up to an hour, but apart from this you may resume normal activities immediately.

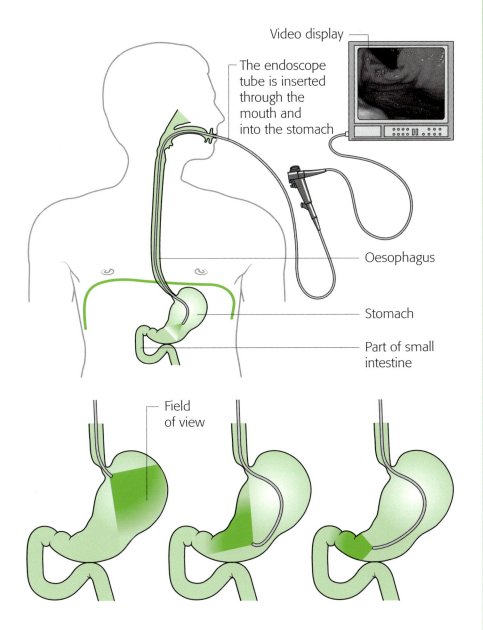

Video display

The endoscope tube is inserted through the mouth and into the stomach

Oesophagus

Stomach

Part of small intestine

Field of view

The endoscope is moved around so that the specialist can examine the lining of the whole stomach and take samples of any areas that appear abnormal

Barium swallow

- A barium swallow is carried out to investigate difficulty in swallowing, or a sensation that food is 'getting stuck' after swallowing. It reveals abnormalities, such as stricture (narrowing), ulcers and hiatus hernia (protrusion of part of the stomach into the chest area), and problems with the movement of food through the oesophagus (gullet).

- The barium swallow is carried out in the X-ray department, and you will be asked not to eat or drink for 6 hours beforehand, so that the picture is clear.

- You will be asked to stand in front of an X-ray video recorder and to swallow a cupful of a special white liquid containing barium, which shows up on the X-ray. You may be given some bread or a marshmallow to eat, as this allows doctors to look at the contractions of muscles in the oesophagus.

- The movement of the oesophagus is filmed continuously during swallowing.

- After the test you may notice chalky white stools for a few days. This is caused by the barium and is harmless.

- You should drink as much fluid as possible for 2–3 days after the procedure to prevent constipation.

- You should receive the results of the investigation within a fortnight.

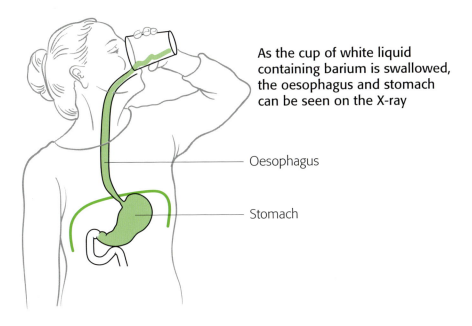

As the cup of white liquid containing barium is swallowed, the oesophagus and stomach can be seen on the X-ray

Oesophagus

Stomach

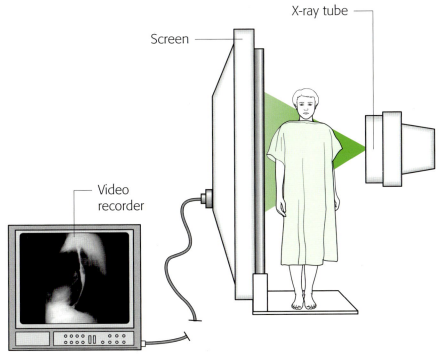

X-ray tube

Screen

Video recorder

Barium meal and follow through

- A barium meal and follow through is used to investigate difficulty in swallowing, abdominal pain and loss of appetite or weight; less often, it is used to diagnose hiatus hernias (protrusion of part of the stomach into the chest area), ulcers, inflammation, cancerous or non-cancerous growths or narrowing of part of the intestines.

- You must eat a low-fibre diet for about 2 days before the investigation to reduce the amount of waste material and gas going through your intestines. The hospital will advise you on what you may eat.

- The day before the test you will be given a strong laxative, which will cause frequent and loose bowel movements. You should drink plenty of fluid during this time to avoid dehydration.

- You must not eat after midnight the night before the test.

- The procedure will take place in the X-ray department. You will be asked to stand in front of an X-ray video recorder and drink a glass of a white liquid containing barium, which is similar to a thick milkshake and shows up on X-ray.

- The progress of the barium will be filmed as you drink the liquid and every 15–30 minutes afterwards. It may take 4 hours or longer for the barium to pass through your intestines.

- After the test you may notice chalky white stools for a few days; this is the barium and is harmless. Drink plenty of fluid for 2 days after the procedure to avoid constipation.

- You should receive the results of the investigation within a fortnight.

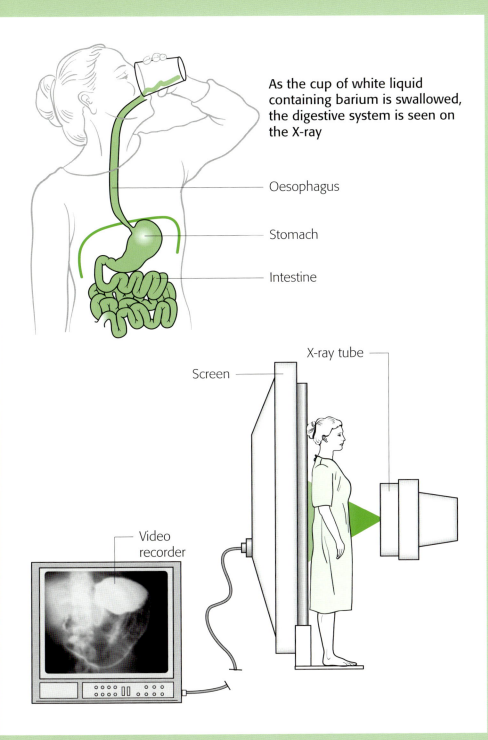

As the cup of white liquid containing barium is swallowed, the digestive system is seen on the X-ray

Oesophagus

Stomach

Intestine

X-ray tube

Screen

Video recorder

Liver biopsy

- A liver biopsy is performed to diagnose and assess inflammation, cirrhosis (liver damage), cancerous and non-cancerous growths and some infections.

- Liver biopsy involves removing a tiny piece of liver tissue using a special needle under a local anaesthetic. Ultrasound may be used to guide the biopsy needle.

- The operation may be carried out as a day case, or you may be admitted to hospital overnight. Blood tests will be arranged beforehand to check that your blood clots normally, in order to minimize the risk of bleeding.

- The biopsy will be taken while you lie comfortably on your back with your right arm resting under your head. The area of skin over your liver will be cleaned to minimize the risk of infection and you will be given an injection of local anaesthetic.

- When the biopsy needle is inserted you will be asked to hold your breath for a few seconds while the sample is taken. This ensures that the liver does not move during the procedure.

- You may feel some discomfort after the procedure, but this will be relieved with painkillers.

- Although bleeding after the biopsy is uncommon, you will be kept under observation for 6 hours as a standard precaution, and your pulse and blood pressure will be checked regularly.

- The tissue sample obtained will be examined in the laboratory. Results are usually available in 1–2 weeks.

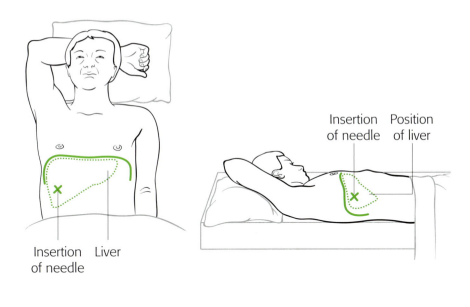

Insertion of needle | Liver

Insertion of needle | Position of liver

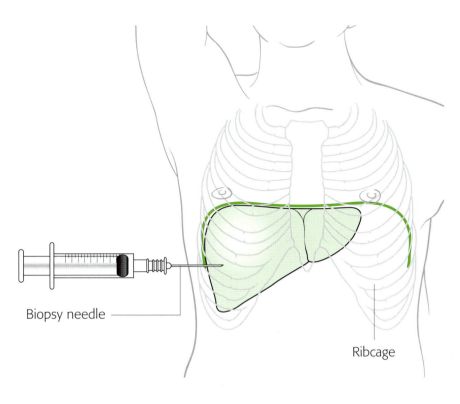

Biopsy needle

Ribcage

Endoscopic retrograde cholangiopancreatography (ERCP)

- Endoscopic retrograde cholangiopancreatography (ERCP) is used to examine the bile ducts, which connect the liver to the small intestine and pancreas. It may be performed if you have jaundice or abdominal pain, or if the doctor suspects that your bile ducts may be blocked (for example, with gallstones).

- You will be asked not to eat or drink for at least 6 hours before the procedure to ensure that your stomach is completely empty.

- Before the test you will be given an injection of a sedative, which will make you drowsy, although you will remain conscious. If there is a risk of infection, such as from a blocked bile duct, you will be given antibiotics.

- A thin, flexible video 'telescope' called an endoscope is passed through the mouth and down into the stomach and the top of the small intestine.

- A dye that is visible on X-ray film is then injected down the endoscope into the bile ducts, and X-rays are taken so that the pancreas and bile ducts can be seen.

- If there are gallstones in the bile duct, they can be caught in a tiny wire basket and removed, and if the duct has narrowed, a stent (a small mesh tube) can be placed in it to hold it open.

- This investigation can be performed as an outpatient procedure, but occasionally it is necessary for patients to stay in hospital overnight for observation.

- You should receive the results of the investigation within a fortnight.

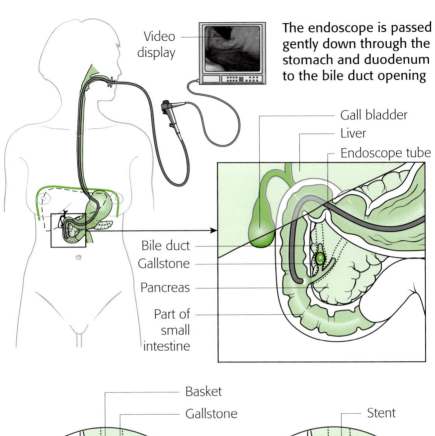

24

Video display

The endoscope is passed gently down through the stomach and duodenum to the bile duct opening

Gall bladder
Liver
Endoscope tube

Bile duct
Gallstone
Pancreas
Part of small intestine

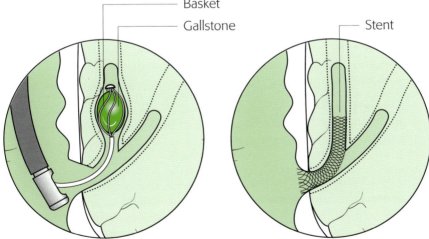

Basket
Gallstone

Stent

Removing gallstones in a wire basket

Widening the bile duct with a stent

Colonoscopy

- Colonoscopy is the examination of the large intestine with a flexible video 'telescope'. It is carried out to investigate bleeding from the rectum (back passage), changes in bowel movements, abdominal pain and abnormalities revealed by other investigations, such as barium enema, to check for disease and to look for polyps (small growths on the wall of the intestine).

- You will be given a laxative on the day before the examination to ensure that your large intestine is empty. From then on you should drink only clear fluids (such as water, black tea or coffee, or squash) to help clean the bowel and avoid dehydration.

- Before the procedure you will be given an injection of sedative, which will make you drowsy, but you will remain conscious.

- For the colonoscopy, you will be asked to lie on your side with your legs drawn up toward your chest. The tube is then passed into the intestine through your rectum.

- Some air will be blown into the intestine during the procedure to improve the view of the intestinal wall. This can make you want to pass wind, and you will be encouraged to do so to reduce any discomfort. Doctors and nurses are used to this, so don't worry.

- The examination is usually performed as an outpatient procedure, and typically lasts 15–30 minutes.

- Occasionally, small pieces of tissue may be removed painlessly (biopsy) by the colonoscope for more detailed examination in the laboratory. Results are usually available in 1–2 weeks. Polyps can also be removed using this procedure.

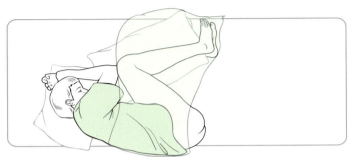

25

Position for colonoscopy

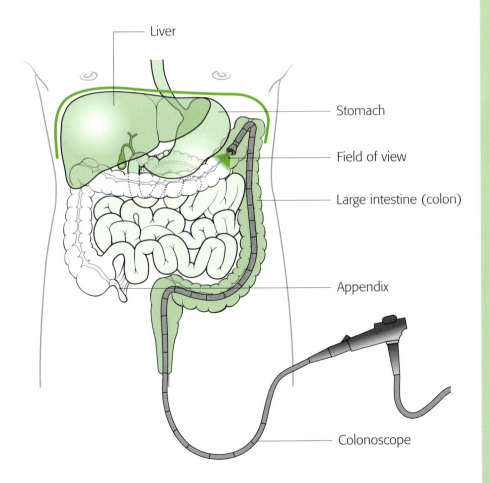

Liver

Stomach

Field of view

Large intestine (colon)

Appendix

Colonoscope

Barium enema

- Barium enema is an X-ray examination of the large intestine and rectum (back passage). It may be performed if you are anaemic or are bleeding from the rectum or you have a change in bowel habit, abdominal pain or diarrhoea.

- The procedure is carried out in the X-ray department and usually lasts 30–60 minutes.

- 2 days before the procedure you will be given a strong laxative that will cause frequent and loose bowel movements, and you will be asked to eat a special low-fibre diet until the barium enema to reduce the amount of waste material and gas going through your intestines. You should drink plenty of clear fluid during this time to avoid dehydration.

- During the procedure you will lie on your left side on a couch with the X-ray camera above you. A tube will then be gently inserted into your rectum. A white liquid containing barium will be passed through this tube, followed by some air, which improves the visibility of the wall of the intestine. You may feel some discomfort during this investigation, but it should not be painful.

- You will be asked to change position during the procedure so that the whole of the large intestine becomes coated with barium and a series of X-ray pictures can be taken.

- After the procedure you may notice chalky white stools for a few days. This is caused by the barium and is harmless. You should drink as much fluid as possible for 2 days after the procedure to avoid constipation.

- You should receive the results of the investigation within a fortnight.

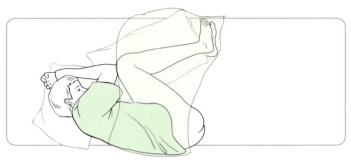

26

Initial position

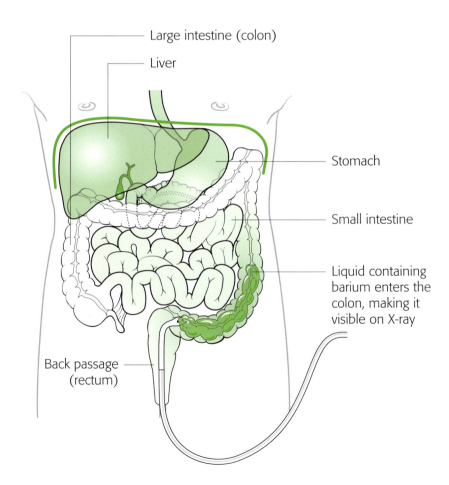

Large intestine (colon)

Liver

Stomach

Small intestine

Liquid containing barium enters the colon, making it visible on X-ray

Back passage (rectum)

Capsule endoscopy

- Because the small bowel is between the stomach and the colon, and is very long, it cannot be fully examined by instruments passed through the mouth or anus.

- Instead, you can swallow a capsule endoscope, which is about 2.5 × 1 cm in size and contains a camera, light, battery and transmitter to send video images.

- Capsule endoscopy may be used when standard endoscopic examinations of the stomach, duodenum and colon have failed to find a cause for conditions such as chronic diarrhoea, anaemia and gastrointestinal bleeding.

- You will be advised in advance what you may eat and drink before capsule endoscopy. The day before, you will be asked to drink clear fluids only after a light breakfast or lunch.

- On the day, sensor leads are taped to your abdomen and you put on a harness holding the recorder before swallowing the capsule. This is easier than swallowing a conventional tablet, as it has a smooth surface, and you will not feel it inside you.

- You can leave the hospital and go about your life with the recording apparatus hidden underneath your clothing. You will be able to drink 2 hours later and eat 4 hours later.

- After about 8 hours, you return to the hospital, and the recorder and sensors will be removed so that the specialists can view the recording. The capsule will be passed naturally in the stools and does not need to be retrieved.

- The procedure is extremely safe, although in rare cases where the small bowel is narrowed, the capsule can be retained. If you have had previous bowel surgery or are thought to be at risk of such a problem you may undergo tests first.

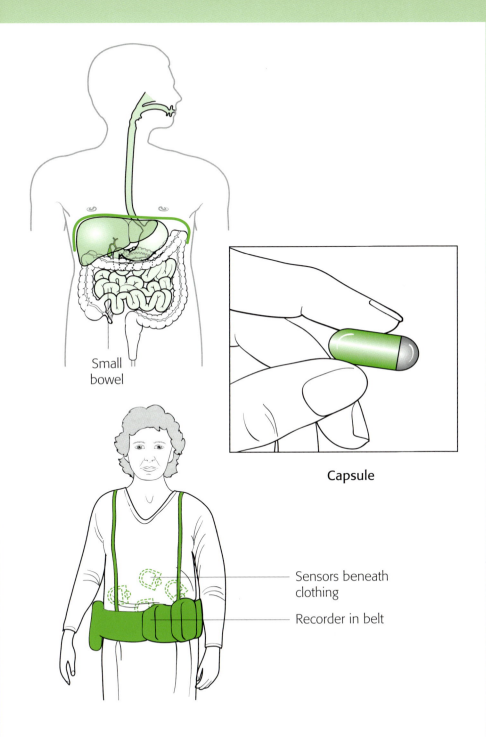

27

Small
bowel

Capsule

Sensors beneath
clothing

Recorder in belt

Dilation of oesophageal stricture

- Stricture (narrowing) of the oesophagus (gullet) causes difficulty in swallowing, or creates the sensation that food is stuck in the throat. It may occur for a variety of reasons.

- The symptoms can be helped by a simple procedure in which the narrowed area of oesophagus is stretched to widen it.

- Before the procedure you will be given painkillers to avoid any discomfort during the stretching, and an injection of sedative. The sedative will cause drowsiness, although you will remain conscious.

- A thin, flexible video 'telescope' called an endoscope is used to insert a fine wire into the narrowed oesophagus. Sometimes X-rays must be used to guide this procedure. The endoscope is then withdrawn and the area stretched using a series of dilators. Alternatively, a small balloon may be gently inflated in the oesophagus. Both procedures take only a few minutes and are normally carried out as day cases in hospital.

- Swallowing is improved immediately, and you will be able to drink 2 hours after the procedure, but you may have a sore throat for a few days.

- After the procedure you will be monitored for some time to check that the oesophagus has not been damaged. You may also have a chest X-ray. In a very small number of patients stretching causes a tear in the oesophagus. This is treated in hospital by either 'resting' the oesophagus and being fed through a drip, or with an operation to repair or remove the affected section.

- If your symptoms return, the procedure can be repeated to increase the width of the oesophagus.

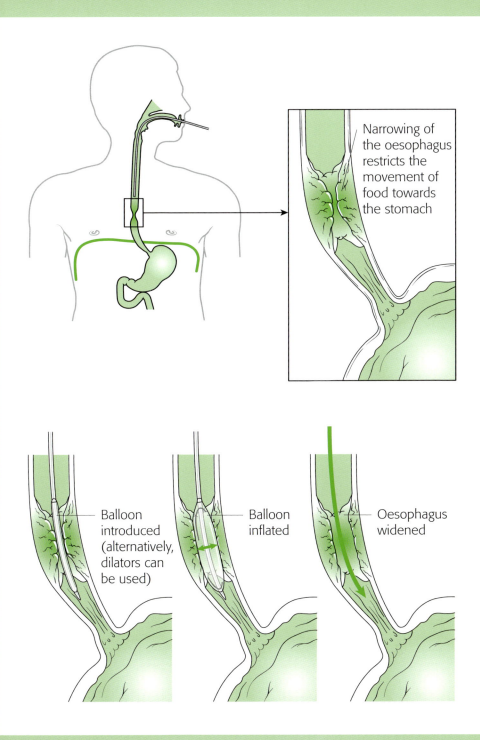

28

Narrowing of the oesophagus restricts the movement of food towards the stomach

Balloon introduced (alternatively, dilators can be used)

Balloon inflated

Oesophagus widened

Insertion of an oesophageal stent

- Narrowing of the oesophagus (gullet) can be treated by inserting an expandable tube, called a stent, made of metal or plastic, which permanently holds the oesophagus open and improves swallowing.

- The stent is inserted using an endoscope – a flexible video 'telescope' – either in the X-ray department or in the endoscopy unit.

- The narrowed area may be dilated (stretched) first, and then the stent is placed into the oesophagus using the endoscope.

- The procedure takes approximately 20 minutes, though you will usually have to stay in hospital for at least one night.

- Swallowing should be improved immediately, although you may have a sore throat for up to 2 days. It is usually recommended that you start with fluids and soft food before progressing back to your normal diet. Once it is in place, you will not be aware of the stent, even when swallowing.

- It is suggested that you have a fizzy drink after eating, as this will help to keep the stent clear of bits of food.

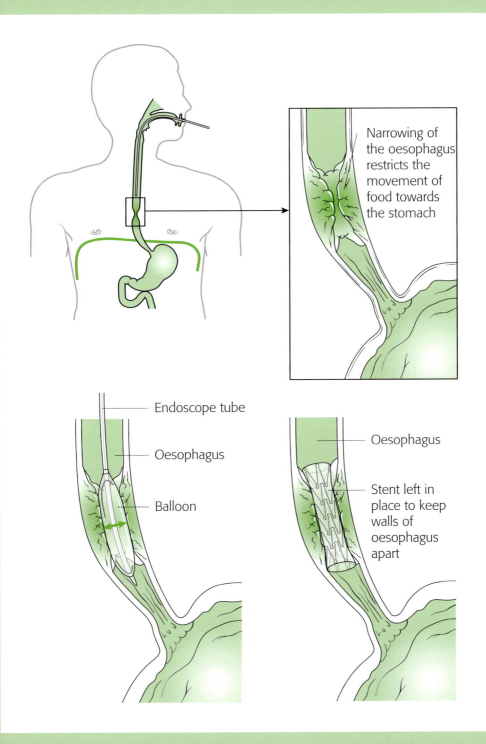

29

Narrowing of the oesophagus restricts the movement of food towards the stomach

Endoscope tube

Oesophagus

Balloon

Oesophagus

Stent left in place to keep walls of oesophagus apart

Injection sclerotherapy and banding of oesophageal varices

- Oesophageal varices are veins under the surface of the oesophagus (gullet) that have become prominent and swollen due to liver damage. As they increase in size, they become more likely to bleed.

- To prevent major blood loss, the varices must be treated immediately. Treatment involves 'shrinking' the varices.

- Injection sclerotherapy and oesophageal banding are techniques that are used to shrink oesophageal varices.

- Injection sclerotherapy involves introducing a needle into the oesophagus through a thin flexible video 'telescope' called an endoscope, and injecting the veins with a fluid which causes them to shrink.

- Alternatively, banding of the varices involves placing a small rubber band around part of the swollen vein, causing it to shrink and die, reducing the size of the vein and leaving a small scar. The band drops off and passes naturally through the digestive tract. This procedure may need to be repeated once or twice.

- Injection sclerotherapy and banding are usually outpatient procedures. They are not painful, although you may feel some discomfort for 24 hours afterwards. After the procedure, you will be able to take liquids; the next day, you may eat soft foods, and on the third day you will be able to eat as normal.

- After all the varices have disappeared, you should have annual checks to ensure that no more have formed.

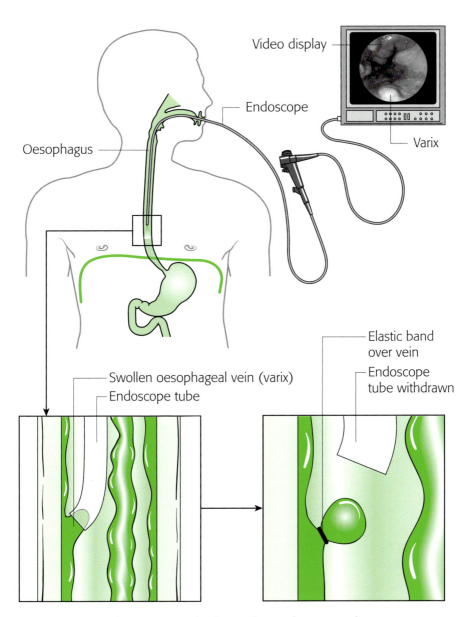

30

Video display

Endoscope

Varix

Oesophagus

Swollen oesophageal vein (varix)

Endoscope tube

Elastic band over vein

Endoscope tube withdrawn

The vein is sucked into the endoscope tube and an elastic band placed on it

Extraction of gallstones at endoscopic retrograde cholangiopancreatography (ERCP)

- Gallstones can be removed from the bile ducts during an investigation, usually for outpatients, called endoscopic retrograde cholangiopancreatography (ERCP).

- Before the procedure you will be given an injection of sedative, which will make you drowsy, but you will remain conscious. You may also be given antibiotics to prevent infection.

- The endoscope, a flexible video 'telescope', is passed gently into the mouth and down into the duodenum (the first part of the small intestine). At the bile ducts, a dye that will be visible on X-rays is injected down the endoscope. X-rays of the pancreas, bile ducts and gall bladder are then taken.

- The gallstones are removed by making a small cut at the entrance to the bile duct and passing a balloon or small wire basket through the endoscope to move the stone into the duodenum. The stone is then excreted with other body waste.

- ERCP may, rarely, cause some bleeding from the bile ducts. If this happens you will need to stay in hospital for treatment.

- Occasionally it is not possible to remove the gallstone(s) with this procedure and an operation is needed.

- It is not possible to remove stones from the gall bladder itself by ERCP, so an operation to remove the gall bladder is often recommended to prevent any recurrence of the problem. This does not have any serious, long-term effects on your health.

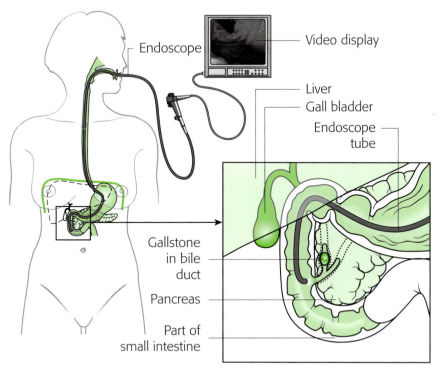

31

Endoscope

Video display

Liver

Gall bladder

Endoscope tube

Gallstone in bile duct

Pancreas

Part of small intestine

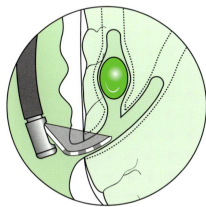

A small cut is made to allow endoscope instruments to be inserted into the bile duct

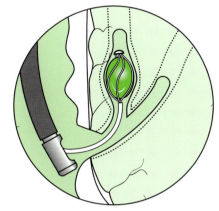

A wire basket attached to the endoscope is used to 'capture' the gallstone and remove it from the bile duct

Useful contacts

CORE (The Digestive Disorders Foundation)
3 St Andrew's Place
London NW1 4LB
www.corecharity.org.uk
info@corecharity.org.uk
Tel: 020 7486 0341
Fax: 020 7224 2012

Cancer BACUP
3 Bath Place
Rivington Street
London EC2A 3JR
www.cancerbacup.org.uk
Helplines: 0808 800 1234
020 7739 2280

CancerHelp UK
Cancer Information Department
Cancer Research UK
PO Box 123
Lincoln's Inn Fields
London WC2A 3PX
www.cancerhelp.org.uk
cancer.info@cancer.org.uk

The Coeliac Society UK
PO Box 220, High Wycombe
Buckinghamshire HP11 2HY
www.coeliac.co.uk
Tel: 01494 437238
Fax: 01494 474349

British Liver Trust
Portman House, 44 High Street
Ringwood, Hampshire BH24 1AG
www.britishlivertrust.org.uk
Tel: 01425 463080
Fax: 01425 470706

National Association for Colitis and Crohn's Disease (NACC)
4 Beaumont House
Sutton Road
St Albans
Hertfordshire AL1 5HH
www.nacc.org.uk
nacc@nacc.org.uk
Tel (information): 0845 130 2233
Tel (support): 0845 130 3344
Tel (administration): 01727 830038
Fax: 01727 862550

IBS Network
Unit 5, 53 Mowbray Street
Sheffield S3 8EN
www.ibsnetwork.org.uk
info@ibsnetwork.org.uk
Tel: 0114 272 3253

Beating Bowel Cancer
39 Crown Road
St Margarets
Twickenham
Middlesex TW1 3EJ
www.bowelcancer.org
info@beatingbowelcancer.org
Tel: 020 8892 5256
Tel (helpline): 020 8892 1331
(Tues 9.30 AM–5PM, Fri 9.00 AM–1PM)
Fax: 020 8892 1008

British Colostomy Association
15 Station Road
Reading
Berkshire RG1 1LG
www.bcass.org.uk
Tel: 0118 939 1537
Fax: 0118 956 9095

British Society of Gastroenterology
3 St Andrew's Place, Regent's Park
London NW1 4LB
www.bsg.org.uk
bsg@mailbox.ulcc.ac.uk
Tel: 020 7387 3534
Fax: 020 7487 3734

**British Association for Parenteral
and Enteral Nutrition**
Secure Hold Business Centre
Studley Road, Redditch
Worcestershire B98 7LG
www.bapen.org.uk

The Helicobacter Foundation
www.helico.com

Mail order

This book is one of a series.

Current *Patient Pictures* titles:
- *Bladder Disorders*
- *Breast Cancer*
- *Cardiology*
- *Ear, Nose and Throat*
- *End-Stage Renal Failure*
- *Erectile Dysfunction*
- *Fertility*
- *Gastroenterology (2nd edition)*
- *Gynaecological Oncology*
- *Gynaecology (2nd edition)*
- *HIV Medicine*
- *Ophthalmology*
- *Prostatic Diseases and their Treatments*
- *Respiratory diseases*
- *Rheumatology (2nd edition)*
- *Urological Surgery*

To order direct using your credit card, call
01752 202301 in the UK, +44 1752 202301 in Europe,
800 266 5564 in the USA or 419 281 1802 in Canada.

For an order form or an up-to-date list of Health Press titles, visit the website
www.patientpictures.com
e-mail us at
post@healthpress.co.uk
or phone or fax:
Tel: +44 (0) 1235 523233
Fax: +44 (0) 1235 523238

Visit our website
www.patientpictures.com